Iara Pantoja
Raely Amorim
Glenda Ferreira

Healthy Communities: Experience through active methodologies

Iara Pantoja
Raely Amorim
Glenda Ferreira

Healthy Communities: Experience through active methodologies

Health promotion strategy

Publisher:
Sciencia Scripts
is a trademark of
Dodo Books Indian Ocean Ltd. and OmniScriptum S.R.L publishing group

120 High Road, East Finchley, London, N2 9ED, United Kingdom
Str. Armeneasca 28/1, office 1, Chisinau MD-2012, Republic of Moldova, Europe
Printed at: see last page
ISBN: 978-620-7-98453-4

SUMMARY

CHAPTER 1

INTRODUCTION

1.1 ON THE SUBJECT UNDER STUDY

The different social spaces are scenes of daily life for individuals, families and communities, and occur in well-defined territories, each with its own local and regional peculiarities, to which health actions and services must be directed in order to meet health needs (BRASIL, 2015). Machado et al. (2007) believe that comprehensive care must perceive the user as a historical, social and political subject, linked to their family context, the environment and the society in which they live. In this way, it becomes important to recognise the individual in their social context.

For priority groups such as the elderly, spaces for social interaction can have an even greater social and health significance, and include homes, schools, long-term care institutions for the elderly (LTCIEs), hostels and crèches. In the case of institutionalised elderly people, LTCIEs have ambiguous meanings, being identified as a place of care and as a place that imprisons and mortifies (OLIVEIRA; ROSENDO, 2014).

To understand institutionalised elderly people, we need to know their life story. It is from knowing the family, social and economic context, experiences, wishes and desires of this population that we can fully meet their care needs (OLIVEIRA; ROSENDO, 2014). In this age group, chronic diseases are more prevalent and require care to be prescribed based on individualised nursing diagnoses (OLIVEIRA et al., 2008; DANTAS et al., 2013).

Social spaces **historically represent important spaces for health practices and experiences present in the relationships between the participants who** live in this scenario, in which determining factors of health and disease conditions can be problematised and analysed (SILVA; BODSTEIN, 2016). The health problems prevalent in elderly individuals are different from those of school-age children (SOUZA et al., 2013).

In LTCFs, care is often fragmented and focussed; therefore, there is an urgent need for comprehensive care that balances clinical care, prevention and health promotion (TEIXEIRA et al., 2014). From this perspective, the work of health professionals must go beyond traditional health institutions such as hospitals, outpatient units and urgent and emergency care centres. Their working methods must also be focused on the individual, eliminating the focus on technicality. As a health professional, nurses can provide their professional care in different spaces, from the traditional to new places of care practice such as the home, schools, community associations, factories, among others (COFEN, 2009).

The practice of this professional in these environments must be carried out deliberately and systematically, using the systematisation of nursing care (SNC), which is organised into five interrelated, interdependent and recurring stages, namely: collection of nursing data or nursing history; nursing diagnosis; planning of nursing care; implementation; and nursing evaluation (COFEN, 2009).

To this end, there is a need to rethink praxis, looking for health promotion practices that can activate the power of action to build measures that result in strengthening participants and collectivities, expanding autonomy and encouraging their participation (MENDES; FERNADEZ, 2016). For health professionals, rethinking praxis for social transformation can sometimes become more complex, requiring a collective effort, using strategies such as continuing education, through meaningful learning (SILVA et al., 2010). From this perspective, training institutions have an important role to play, because as Goulart (2004) points out, education has a transformative role to play in the formation of conscious participants and authentic citizens (GOULART, 2004). So that they can equip participants to transform their living conditions in their various social spaces.

In order for reality to be transformed, by changing the professional praxis and the participants, through action-research activities, considering this as a learning mechanism, which is why it is inextricably linked to teaching and research (GOULART, 2004). To achieve this goal, action research is a viable methodological approach, since it is an empirical process that identifies the problem within a social and/or institutional context, carries out data collection, followed by the analysis and signification of the data collected by the participants. In addition to identifying the need for change and identifying possible solutions (KOERICH et al., 2009).

1. 2 JUSTIFICATION

Spaces such as LTCIEs are frequented by individuals from priority groups, with different health conditions that require health professionals to adopt innovative practices in these spaces of daily life.

Recognising these environments as non-traditional places for providing care and, above all, guidance for self-care practices is a field to be better explored by health professionals, who should look for unconventional practices to intervene in the health needs of these groups, based on the construction of care plans that facilitate assistance and health promotion, as a strategy for health and social intervention, aimed at emancipating the individual in self-care and care practices.

In this context, considering intervention in practice in order to bring about transformation, it is necessary to use methodological tools, which include our own methods of care and methods that are capable of combining theory and practice experienced in academia; SAE and action research fulfil these functions, respectively.

In order to use two methods that differ in their purpose, but have a single end goal, which is the transformation of a given reality, we sought to bring academia closer to people's everyday lives, in an understanding of the individual as a singular subject who interacts, and as a subject who is part of a collectivity.

In this way, new perspectives on the health panorama can be produced. Among the multiplicity of methodological approaches, action research emerged both as a tool for including participants and as a possibility for transforming health practices. We believe this is an important methodology because it combines research and action simultaneously, i.e. academia and practice as a two-way street.

The extension activities experienced by students during their academic life awaken their clinical competence, resulting in a process of cognitive, psychomotor and affective development that makes them better able to assess, plan, implement and evolve care for individuals, families and communities, as well as the environment in which they live. These skills are expected by the labour market, which is looking for professionals with innovative and creative initiatives.

1.3 PROBLEM SITUATION

In Brazil, there has been a change in public health policies in recent years, with micro-territories being considered as privileged spaces for intervention, since these are where individuals establish their relationships and where the health-disease process takes place (BRASIL, 2015).

In Brazil, ILPIs are often philanthropic, small and house around 30 residents. They are home to around 100,000 people, with a predominance of women (57.3 per cent) among the residents (CAMARANO; KANSO, 2010). For Freitas and Noronha (2010, p. 360), they represent **"privileged places to observe this way of** living old age, being a scenario full of different life stories, marked **by negative and positive impressions about the meaning of being elderly"**.

According to Dantas (2013), the situations that lead family members to hospitalise their elderly loved ones in long-term care institutions are due to abandonment, difficulty in dealing with and caring for the elderly person who has a vascular, metabolic or mental illness, as well as domestic violence. In addition, these circumstances can develop risks that affect the emotional and physical structure of these people, such as loneliness, malnutrition, falls and skin lesions (MOREIRA, 2014).

In order to work in these non-traditional care spaces, health professionals must transform their practices beyond technicality. The literature describes that the care provided by professionals to the elderly does not always correspond to what is expected of them, and there is a need to further explore the issue of the elderly in long-term care institutions and the care provided to them (FREITAS; NORONHA, 2010).

In this way, the involvement of professional nurses with the use of the nursing process in these environments is called nursing consultation and is indispensable (COFEN, 2009). The applicability of systematised nursing care (SNC) in institutionalised elderly people is necessary in order to make diagnoses based on the identification of problems and risks that can interfere with the quality of life of these individuals (DIAS, 2014; PIRES et al., 2012).

Despite this, this method of working is rarely applied outside the institutions where health care has historically taken place, and is even unknown to nursing professionals (SILVA; GARCEZ; PESTANA, 2010). In order to operationalise SNC, it is necessary to overcome paradigm shifts in thinking, being and acting (VARELA et al., 2012).

Considering that the proposal presented is an action research project, the essence of which is to establish a connection between the theory built up in the classroom and the practice experienced in the academy, the aim is to equip students through active methodologies to integrate the various disciplines of the course.

Considering that nurses can use the SNC to provide comprehensive care that gives patients and their families a better quality of life, they can identify their real needs and make direct interventions through care planning (FURTADO; NÓBREGA; FONTES, 2007). In view of the above, we reflected on the need to utilise SNC applied to participants in non-traditional care settings. Faced with this problem, we question some aspects:

Are the health conditions of the elderly adequate?

Are the health conditions of the elderly inadequate?

1.4 OBJECTIVES

1.4.1. General Objective

Evaluating the health conditions of elderly people living in ILPIs in Belém, Pa.

1.4.2. Specific objectives

- Describe the epidemiological profile of the study population;
- To find out about the daily living habits of elderly people living in an ILPI in Belém;
- To know the inspection and evaluation of the cranial nerve pairs of the study population.

CHAPTER 2

THEORETICAL REFERENCE

Ageing is a phase marked by physiological, physical, psychological and social changes. It is part of the life cycle and is an irreversible process (MACIEL, 2007 apud CARREIRA, 2010). The elderly in Brazil age in a heterogeneous way, when taking into account functionality, control of diseases and illnesses, accessibility to health services, support network and lifestyle (DIAS, 2014).

According to the 2010 demographic census, the number of people over 65 in Brazil is 14,081,480 million, equivalent to 7.6 per cent of the population, with 3.4 per cent men and 4.2 per cent women (IBGE, 2011). It has been estimated that in two decades - 2000 to 2020 - life expectancy for men will increase to 70 years and for women to 76 years. By 2050, 38 million Brazilians will be over 65. This data points to an increase in women's longevity, which may be related to lifestyle (CHAIMOWICZ, 2013).

Considering the profile of the elderly population in Brazil, studies in various cities in different regions have identified a predominance of females, aged between 60 and 70, with low income and schooling. As for marital status, in the southeast there is a higher frequency of single elderly people, while in some cities in other regions married/widowed marital status prevailed. In a study carried out in the North and Northeast, it was found that the elderly have more children, on average 6, while in the South and Southeast the average is 2 children (MIRANDA et al., 2016; CLARES et al., 2011; CAUDURO et al., 2011; SUDRÉ et al., 2014).

In long-term care institutions for the elderly (LTCIEs), the vast majority are single, poorly educated individuals without children, who generally seek institutionalisation for health treatment. Along with this, there is also the family's inability to care for the elderly or to find someone to take responsibility for this care (ALENCAR et al., 2012).

According to studies in various ILPIs in the regions of Brazil, there is a predominance of females, except in the Centre West region. Most of the elderly residents are over 70, illiterate and single. In the Centre West region, the elderly carry out their daily activities independently of help, while in the North most were dependent on help to carry out their daily actions (LISBOA, CHIANCA, 2012; PINHEIRO et al., 2016; OLIVEIRA, NOVAES, 2013; SMANIOTO, HADDAD, 2011; POLARO et al., 2012).

2.2 ELDERLY RESIDENTS OF LONG-STAY INSTITUTIONS

Long-stay institutions for the elderly (ILPI) are specialised homes that provide continuous care for elderly residents. They should be places with the characteristics of a home, a place that brings comfort, security and tranquillity, and should not be characterised by isolation (SILVA, 2010).

Some of the objectives of ILPIs are to re-establish or maintain health conditions and the functional capacity of their residents, as well as to plan and carry out care and educational activities aimed at preventing physical and mental dependence in the group (BARROS, 2010; BORGES, 2015).

They need to be residential, may or may not be governmental and should promote quality of life. One factor that can lead to greater demand for ILPIs is the reduced availability of support and family insufficiency (BORGES, 2015; DANTAS, 2013).

According to Camarano and Kanso (2010), most institutions for the elderly are philanthropic and women predominate. Brazilian institutions live essentially off the resources provided by residents and/or family members, as well as their own resources. In another study, the majority were depressed, they were women, the predominant marital status was single followed by widowed, and around half of those interviewed were taking antidepressant medication (CARREIRA et al, 2011).

The study by Oliveira and Rozendo (2014) identified three functions of ILPIs, according to the elderly. For the first, the needs are food, hygiene, housing and rest. The second function refers to elderly people who have become institutionalised in order to improve and/or maintain their health, since some elderly people report needing assistance and this was the main motivation for institutionalisation. As for the third function, the reports of the elderly people surveyed reveal that they are institutionalised because they treat the ILPIs as a family context and find protection in their staff and, due to family insufficiency, prefer to grow old and die in an ILPI.

The study by Pinheiro et al. (2015), which compares for-profit and non-profit long-term care institutions, reveals that the main reasons for institutionalisation for residents of non-profit institutions were: **family** conflicts **and abandonment, while in for-profit institutions the main reason was "being ill". In the non-profit institutions, more than 90 per cent of the sample did not have** health insurance, while in the for-profit institutions, more than 85 per cent had health insurance. This study reveals the disparity between institutions.

A large proportion of the elderly resort to an ILPI out of resignation, with the aim of reducing the difficulties they face in their daily lives due to the evolution of ageing (OLIVEIRA, ROZENDO, 2014). The loss of functional capacity and the search for quality of life is one of the risk factors for institutionalisation (ALENCAR et al., 2012). Another risk factor is the lack of stimulation provided by some ILPIs, which can be a trigger for a reduction in the potential for autonomy and dependence of some elderly people, interfering with their quality of life as they grow older (BARROS, 2010).

The multidisciplinary team in an ILPI should aim to promote autonomy and independence, as well as encouraging self-care in each elderly resident (CLARES, 2013). In particular, nursing professionals must meet the basic needs of the elderly, as they are directly responsible for the care provided to ILPI residents (CASTRO, 2015). Nurses must be qualified in their care for the elderly due to the complexity of events such as frailty, dependency, clinical conditions and the risk of complications (DANTAS, 2013). As well as providing social, emotional and affective support, benefiting the health and well-being of elderly residents of ILPIs (BORGES, 2015).

2.3 NURSING CARE FOR THE ELDERLY

2.3.1. Health condition of the elderly

Brazil's demographic profile is rapidly progressing towards a demographic transition, in which it is characterised by an ageing process that is growing in proportion to the expansion of chronic diseases (MENDES, 2011).

A study analysing health and safety indicators in the elderly revealed a higher prevalence of pressure injuries and falls with injuries. Pressure injuries are a major problem in the lives of the elderly, and they can be avoided with early identification of risk factors and the implementation of preventative measures (CAVALCANTE, 2016).

According to Pereira et al. (2015), their study analysing pain in institutionalised elderly people showed that more than 75% of the elderly in their study had been living with pain for six months or more. The survey was divided into global pain, pain at rest and pain on movement. With regard to overall pain, the majority classify it as severe, at rest and the classification of no pain was used more often by the participants in the survey, while when moving, severe pain appears again more frequently. For the author, there are conceptions that pain is part of the ageing process, a fact that prevents proper pain management.

One of the most common complaints in the elderly population is dizziness, which can give the impression of an imminent fall, instability or vertigo. A study carried out in Rio Grande do Sul revealed that 48.9 per cent of the elderly sample had dizziness during the survey. The average number of associated illnesses was 4.5. The average number of medications per elderly person was 7.8, with the maximum number of medications being 17. The same study found that 29.2% of elderly people with dizziness had a fracture due to a fall (ROSA et al., 2016).

With regard to falls, extrinsic factors stand out, such as inadequate flooring, lighting, stairs and physical barriers in general. Most elderly people who have already suffered falls develop a fear of falling again, which creates a risk of physical inactivity and worsening balance. A study carried out in the Federal District revealed that 79.8 per cent of the elderly had fallen, 65.1 per cent of them from their own height, with contusion and fracture being the most common injuries (FREITAS, 2015).

The most common chronic diseases in the elderly are heart disease, cerebrovascular disease, diabetes, lung diseases related to smoking, pneumonia, neoplasms and transport accidents (CHAIMOWICZ, 2013). In addition to these diseases, Oliveira and Novaes (2013) identified gastrointestinal and joint problems. In relation to morbidities, according to Miranda, Soares and Silva (2016), the most common among the elderly are hypertension, dyslipidaemia, diabetes mellitus and osteoarticular diseases. Most elderly people have at least one type of chronic disease (ALENCAR et al., 2012).

According to studies by Garbaccio and Ferreira (2012), in a long-stay institution, the most prominent diseases identified were: hypertension, diabetes mellitus, hypothyroidism, alcoholic neuropathy, heart disease, musculoskeletal diseases, prostate/breast cancer, renal failure/liver failure, hyperthyroidism, Parkinson's disease, epilepsy, chronic obstructive pulmonary disease and Chagas disease.

Despite the longevity of this population, there is a presence of comorbidities and chronic non-communicable diseases, consequently causing greater functional incapacity, which is one of the main geriatric syndromes (MARCHON, 2010; MORAES et al., 2010).

The health of the elderly is related to overall functionality, i.e. being able to manage their own lives and take care of themselves, and these abilities are measured by the analysis of daily life, which assesses autonomy and independence. Several studies have used this analysis to find out about the functional performance of the elderly (MORAES et al., 2010; DANTAS et al., 2013; FUHRMANN, 2015).

Functional capacity is determined as the physical and mental ability to lead an independent and autonomous life (MARCHON, 2010). According to Moraes et al. (2010), the domains of the elderly are characterised by functionality, having the ability to function on their own. These functions are assessed through the Activities of Daily Living (ADLs), which for the elderly to carry them out require the individual's predisposition to make decisions, called autonomy, and independence, which is the ability to do something by their own specific means. These areas are determined by the harmonious functioning of four functional domains: cognition, mood, mobility and communication (Figure 1). The loss of these functions triggers the main geriatric syndromes: cognitive incapacity, postural instability, immobility and communicative incapacity.

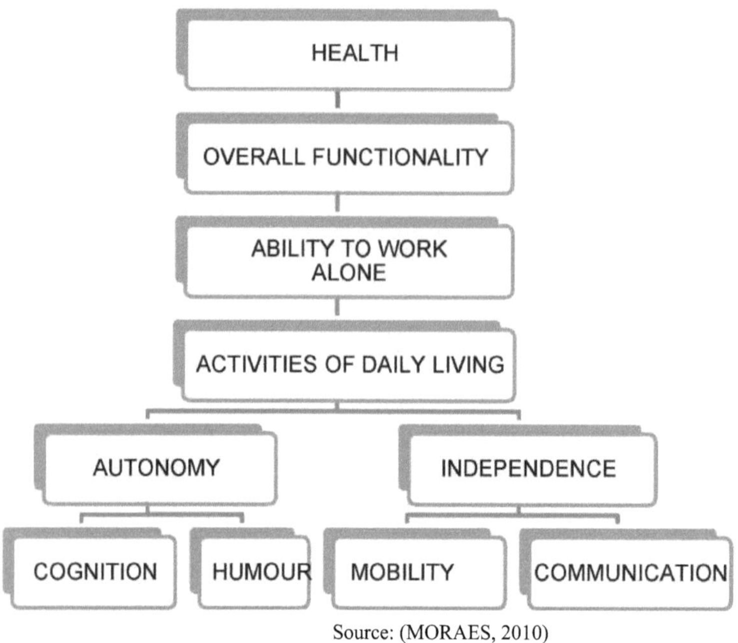

Source: (MORAES, 2010)

According to Dias (2014), the performance of ADLs are parameters for determining an individual's functional status. They can be divided into Basic Activities of Daily Living (BADL), Instrumental Activities of Daily Living (IADL) and Advanced Activities of Daily Living (AADL). The Katz index assesses BADLs, which analyse the activities of bathing, dressing, toileting, transferring, continence and feeding. The scale proposed by Lawton and Brody in 1969 refers to IADLs. This scale includes eight activities: using the telephone, shopping, preparing meals, cleaning, doing laundry, using transport, taking medication and managing finances. The AADLs are classified into social, productive, physical and leisure activities, the main ones being manual labour, hobbies, intellectual and relaxation activities and religious activities.

Independence is characterised so that self-care is possible. A study carried out in Brasilia found that 77% of the institutionalised elderly in the sample had some dependence when it came to carrying out Activities of Daily Living (ADLs), while 23% were independent (LISBOA, 2012).

The quality of life of the institutionalised elderly reveals that, in their view, quality of life is having good health, living in peace and being useful, carrying out their tasks without the help of others and in a cheerful way brings satisfaction to the residents, which shows that autonomy and independence are linked to quality of life (LIMA et al., 2016).

Fuhrmann's (2015) study on the functional capacity of the elderly revealed that the average age in the study was 81.41 years. Most had severe dependence, requiring partial or total help with activities of daily living.

In his study, Duca (2011) highlighted the prevalence of functional incapacity in at least one Activity of Daily Living (ADL) was 79.4%, with 40% of the sample revealing five or six ADLs with functional incapacity. 61.6% of the elderly needed the help of a carer. The sample was again predominantly female. Independence to eat was the most frequent, while independence to bathe was the least frequent.

The study by Barros (2010) reveals that the most dependent Activities of Daily Living were bathing and feeding, while transference and continence were less representative. As age advances, so does the degree of dependence on these functions.

2.3.2. Systematisation of Nursing Care

Considering that the systematisation of nursing care should be used wherever nursing care is provided, it consists of several stages that begin with the nursing history, followed by the nursing diagnosis and nursing interventions or prescriptions, and finally the expected results (COFEN, 2009).

The application of SNC must be based on a theoretical model of care. In Brazil, the adoption of theoretical models to guide professional practice, both in care and teaching, began with Horta's theory of basic human needs (FURTADO, 2007; BARROS, 2009).

Organising and systematising actions are inherent to human beings so that goals/results can be achieved. This method, if devoid of theoretical references, does not make it possible to ascertain the phenomena observed by nurses in their daily practice (diagnoses) and the results (outcomes) of their actions (interventions)

(BARROS, 2009).

In this context, Horta's Basic Human Needs Theory is a theoretical framework that focuses on care centred on meeting the affected needs of the individual, family and community, which provided a broad spectrum of applicability, given that these needs are common to all human beings, differing only in their manifestation and the way they are met, which vary from individual to individual (LOUREIRO, 2006).

According to research by Lira et al, (2015), the most recurrent nursing diagnoses are those of risk and those associated with the respiratory system, locomotion, gastrointestinal system and perception, among them: risk of infection; risk of falls; disturbed sensory perception: vision; fear; pain; altered urinary elimination pattern; risk of unbalanced nutrition less than body needs; impaired physical mobility; impaired gas exchange; altered intestinal elimination pattern; risk of impaired skin integrity; ineffective breathing pattern and excess fluid volume.

Oliveira et al. (2011) identified, in addition to the above diagnoses, others that are more prevalent in the elderly such as: chronic pain; constipation; risk of loneliness; risk of unstable glycaemia; impaired oral mucosa; impaired swallowing; insomnia; risk of impaired liver function; diarrhoea; disturbed sensory perception; unbalanced nutrition beyond bodily needs; chronic sadness; impaired tissue integrity; impaired memory and impaired verbal communication (Oliveira et al., 2011).

In elderly residents of an ILPI, the most relevant nursing diagnoses found were: disposition to increased religiosity; impaired gas exchange; impaired dentition; risk of falls; impaired ambulation; deficit in self-care for dressing; impaired skin integrity; impaired memory; unbalanced nutrition: more than bodily needs; impaired verbal communication; risk of infection; chronic pain; disturbed sensory perception: auditory; risk of impaired skin integrity; unbalanced nutrition: less than bodily needs; disturbed sensory perception: visual; constipation; impaired bed mobility; ineffective peripheral tissue perfusion; anxiety and acute pain (GARBACCIO, FERREIRA, 2012).

Lira et al. (2015) implemented the most relevant nursing prescriptions according to the diagnoses proposed in their study of hospitalised elderly people. These were related to fall prevention, skin integrity, diet and elimination care, risk of falls, respiratory care, mobilisation and water intake.

In studies carried out in the north-east of Brazil, nursing care was developed according to the needs assessed in the elderly, defined according to the diagnoses obtained. This was mainly characterised by medication control, environmental control, ambulation, self-care assistance, fall prevention, counselling, patient contact, pain control, reality orientation, anxiety reduction and memory training (SANTOS et al., 2012).

The patient's degree of dependence is one of the determining factors for nursing care, which is proportional to the increase in the patient's degree of dependence when carrying out activities of daily living. The main interventions found in hospitalised elderly patients were: changing position, assisting with ambulation, bathing and intimate hygiene, identifying the presence of pain, indicating its location and intensity, and observing and communicating behavioural, motor and sensory changes (LUCCHESI, FERRETTI-REBUSTINI, 2015).

In order to offer the elderly adequate, safe and ethical care, it is necessary to create and implement public policies aimed at the well-being of this segment of the population. In addition to training professionals to care for institutionalised elderly people (LISBOA, 2012).

CHAPTER 3

METHODOLOGY

3.1 TYPE OF STUDY

This study is part of the research and extension project entitled "Healthy **communities**: Professional experience of praxis through active methodologies as a **health promotion strategy**" at UNAMA, funded by the Institute for the Development of the Amazon Foundation (FIDESA). This is an action-research project, which used quantitative and qualitative techniques to analyse the data collected. According to SOARES; CORDEIRO and CAMPOS (2013, p. A173), action research is a methodological modality that

> is essential for nursing, showing that, like any social practice, nursing has the motivation to change, based on the contradictions of health practice, to develop critical/innovative praxis that articulates theory and practice and responds to the health needs of different social groups.

Corroborating the authors, Toledo (2014) states that the emergence of action research is associated not only with a situation of dissatisfaction with classic research paradigms and methods, but also with the need to promote greater articulation between theory and practice in the production of knowledge, through the direct involvement of social groups in understanding and finding solutions to their problems, especially those of a complex nature.

According to Goulart (2004), action research is a great area in **which to produce knowledge, from a perspective in which the student can come "into contact** with the world around him and it is through this reality that he can complement his **learning, intelligencing, that is, reading inside what is in front of him". In order for this to happen, "it is necessary to see extension activities as** a teaching process and not simply as an out-of-school event in which **students go out into the community to provide services". (GOULART, 2004, p. 71).**

3.2 STUDY SITE

***C* Casa de Longa Permanência para idosos São Vicente Paulo: Address:** Tv.
Mauriti, 1061 - Pedreira, Belém - PA, 66093-180. **Telephone:** (91) 3226-4984.

3.3 STUDY PARTICIPANTS

- Twenty-one elderly women living in the São Vicente de Paulo shelter took part in the study.

3.3.1   Inclusion criteria

- Elderly residents of the São Vicente de Paulo shelter, who were conscious and orientated, agreed to take part in the study and signed the Informed Consent Form (ICF - Appendix A).

3.3.2   Exclusion criteria

- Elderly women who were not residents of the St Vincent de Paul shelter,
- Elderly women living in the shelter who were conscious and disorientated or who did not agree to take part in the study and did not sign the Informed Consent Form.

3.4 DATA COLLECTION PERIOD

Data collection took place between 1 August and 16 October 2017.

3.5 DATA COLLECTION INSTRUMENTS AND DATA COLLECTION STRATEGIES

An anamnesis and physical examination script was applied to the elderly (Appendix B). The interview script contains closed and open questions that were applied by the researchers. These questions contain socio-demographic information and information about the participants' daily life habits. A standardised physical examination script adapted from Amante; Rosetto and Schneider (2008) was used to carry out the physical examination of the elderly, in which basic non-invasive physical examination techniques were applied in order to get to know the health conditions of the study population. In an environment that guaranteed privacy, two assistant researchers supervised the researcher in charge of the project.

We also applied the script for 1ª nursing consultation multifunctional assessment of the elderly (Appendix C).

Based on the problems identified in the anamnesis, the main nursing diagnoses applied to the elderly were identified and care and self-care guidance and health promotion practices were prescribed.

So it was done:

A To avoid participants having to spend money on transport;

The application of a pilot test - to validate the adapted form;

R The nursing consultation was carried out and the Informed Consent Form was signed;

R Individualised and group consultations for guidance on self-care.

Evaluating the results of health promotion practices.

After filling in all the fields on the form, the information was entered into a database on a computer, which helped to interpret the data and produce the results.

3.6 DATA PROCESSING AND ANALYSIS

The information was stored in a spreadsheet in the SPSS programme (Excel 2007 - version 12.0.4518.1014) to fill in all the information collected, of whatever nature. Prevalence and other frequencies were calculated using the classic concept of descriptive epidemiology of the number of people.

To analyse nutritional status, the Body Mass Index (BMI) was used, obtained by the interaction of anthropometric measurements of body weight (Kg) and height (m), self-reported in the data collection instrument. These measurements were transcribed into an SPSS spreadsheet and the results obtained using the formula:

$$BMI = \frac{Weight}{Height^2}$$

(ABESO 2016)

3.7 ETHICAL ASPECTS

In terms of ethics, the project was sent to the study site with a letter requesting authorisation for data collection (Appendix C).

After authorisation, the research project was registered on the Brazil Platform and submitted to the UNAMA CCBS Research Ethics Committee (CEP). After approval by the CEP, the researchers forwarded the opinion to the data collection site to schedule the activities. The guidelines and norms of Resolution 466/12 of the National Health Council (CNS) were respected. The research was approved by means of opinion no. 2.218.930.

3.8 RISKS AND BENEFITS

The participants were not subjected to any treatment and/or experimentation using biological samples, only data on their condition was collected through non-invasive practices, nor were any practices used that interfere with health, psychological, social or religious aspects. The identification of problems made it possible to provide health promotion guidelines and self-care techniques, but did not pose any physical, biological or psychosocial risks.

The risks to which the research participants were exposed may have been the disclosure of their names. However, as a strategy to minimise the risks and guarantee the anonymity and confidentiality of the data, when referring to the elderly, they were identified with alphanumeric codes (Id01, Id02).

The data collection instruments will remain in the possession of the researcher responsible for one year and will then be destroyed. In order to preserve the anonymity and confidentiality of each individual's information, in accordance with the guidelines and standards of the National Health Council (CNS). Thus, preserving the identity, privacy and confidentiality of the data of the people involved.

The benefits of the research consist of improving the quality of life of the participants involved, since they have received guidance for self-care both individually and in groups, which will have an impact on their daily lives. In addition, the dissemination of the results will provide benefits for expanding the use of the SNC in non-traditional environments, as a tool for nursing decision-making in the context of providing quality care.

3.9 SUSPENSION OR CLOSURE CRITERIA

This research will not be carried out without the approval of the ethics committee of the University of Amazonia and the management of the study site. The research may be suspended, even after approval, at any time before the deadline stipulated in the schedule in the following cases:

C If the research focuses on any topic other than the one that it has agreed to with this Ethics Committee.

C If it goes beyond the date specified in its realisation schedule.

CHAPTER 4

RESULTS

The participants were 21 elderly people, all of whom were female. Table 1 describes the sociodemographic characteristics of the elderly ILPI residents.

In terms of age, 42.9% (9) were between 87 and 96 years old. With regard to the number of children, the majority, 61.9% (13) have no children, while 9.5% (2) have two children.

When it comes to receiving a pension, 100% of the participants (21) receive the benefit. Regarding the length of time they have lived in the shelter, 71.4% (15) have lived there for 1-10 years, 23.8% (5) for 11-20 years and 4.8% (1) for 21-30 years.

Table 1 - Socio-demographic characteristics of elderly residents in ILPI, <u>Belém-Pará, 2017.</u>

Features sociodemographic	n	%
Age group		
67-76	3	14,3
77-86	8	38,1
87-96	9	42,9
No information	1	4,8
Number of children		
0	13	61,9
1	6	28,6
2	2	9,5
Retirement		
Yes	21	100,0
No	0	
Length of time living in the shelter		
1-10	15	71,4
11-20	5	23,8
21-30	1	4,8

Table 2 shows the distribution of the daily lifestyle habits of the elderly residents of the ILPI. With regard to the number of meals, 85.7 per cent (18) ate more than three meals a day.

With regard to dietary restrictions, 80.9% (17) had no restrictions whatsoever.

In terms of water consumption, 42.9% (9) drink more than five (5) glasses of water a day. When it comes to physical activity, 66.7% (14) do some kind of activity.

With regard to chronic illnesses, it can be seen that musculoskeletal disorders are more frequent in 28.6% (6) of the participants in the survey, although the same number reported not having any chronic illnesses.

It is also possible to highlight the number of elderly people with hypertension and diabetes, 19% (4) of whom appear frequently in the survey. When it comes to participants who take medication on a daily basis, this rises to 81 per cent (17).

Considering the appearance of the skin, 57.1% (12) moisturised every day, while 23.8% (5) never moisturised. 61.9% (13) of the population studied did not need help with daily activities. The majority of participants reported falling, around 76.2% (16) of the elderly, and 66.7% (14) frequently experienced pain.

Table 2 - Distribution of the daily lifestyle habits of the elderly living in ILPI, Belém-Pará, 2017.

Lifestyle habits		n	%
Meals			
	2	1	4,8
	3	2	9,5
>4		18	85,7
Food restriction			
	No	17	80,9
	Yes	4	19,0
Glasses of water during the day			
	1 a 3	5	23,8
	4 a 5	7	33,3
	More than 5	9	42,9
Physical activity			
	No	7	33,3
	Yes	14	66,7
Chronic illness			
	Diabetes	1	4,8
Diabetes and hypertension		4	19,0
	Hypertension	2	9,5
	Rheumatism	1	4,8
	Neurological	1	4,8
	Osteomuscular	6	28,6
	No	6	28,6
Use of medication			

	No	4	19,0
	Yes	17	81,0
Moisturising the skin			
	Daily	12	57,1
	Never	5	23,8
	Weekly	3	14,3
	No answer	1	4,8
Help with activities			
	No	13	61,9
	Yes	8	38,1
Fall			
	No	5	23,8
	Yes	16	76,2
Pain			
	No	6	28,6
	Yes	14	66,7
	No answer	1	4,8

Table 3 shows the distribution of the characteristics observed in the inspection of elderly residents in ILPI, 2017. Regarding the inspection of the scalp, it was assessed whether it was intact, with alopecia, dermatitis, seborrhoea, there was a higher frequency of elderly people with intact scalp 76% (16), however it was found that 10% (2) of the population studied had dermatitis and the same amount had seborrhoea. Alopecia was present in 5% (1) of the elderly.

The eyes were inspected to see if the tear duct was congested, if there was eyelid oedema, if there was a change in vision, pallor of the conjunctiva and other alterations. It was found that 67% (14) had no alterations, while 14% (3) had eyelid oedema. As for the other alterations, 5% (1) of the participants had a congested tear duct, altered vision and pallor of the conjunctiva, as well as other alterations.

The inspection of the nose assessed whether the elderly had a runny nose or an obstructed nose. The inspection revealed that 86% (18) of the population studied had no alterations in this aspect, but 10% (2) had a runny nose at the time of the physical examination and only 5% (1) had an obstructed nose.

The inspection of the mouth assessed the absence of teeth, the presence of broken teeth/halitosis, teeth compatible with age and whether they had dentures. It was found that 62% (13) had dentures, while 5% (1) had each of these alterations.

On inspection of the feet, 29% (6) had oedema. Calluses appeared in 10% (2)

of the population, and onychomycosis/halux valgus was also found in 5% (1) of the research subjects. The study found that 67% (14) had intact skin and 24% (5) had spots.

Table 3 - Distribution of the characteristics observed in the inspection of elderly ILPI residents, 2017.

Inspection	n	%
Scalp Inspection		
Whole	16	76%
Alopecia	1	5%
Dermatitis	2	10%
Seborrhoea	2	10%
Eye Inspection		
Congested left lagrimal canal	1	5%
Eyelid oedema	3	14%
No vision in the left eye	1	5%
Others	1	5%
Pallor of the conjuctiva	1	5%
No change	14	67%
Nose Inspection		
Runny nose	2	10%
Obstruction	1	5%
No change	18	86%
Mouth Inspection		
Absence of teeth	1	5%
Broken teeth/halitosis	1	5%
Teeth compatible with age	2	10%
Dental prosthesis	13	62%
No change	4	19%
Foot Inspection		
Calluses	2	10%
Oedema	6	29%
Cracks	1	5%
Cracks/ Edema	2	10%
Vacant hallux	2	10%
Onychomycosis / Hallux valgus	1	5%
No change	7	34%
Skin Integrity		
Haematoma	1	5%
Stain	5	24%
Stains and blisters	1	5%
Full skin	14	67%

Table 4 shows the information collected during the physical examination of the research subjects, and presents the assessment of the cranial nerve pairs. The first pair of cranial nerves is the olfactory nerve. When assessed, we found a frequency of 75% (15) present, while 10% had total anosmia. With regard to cranial nerves II (Facial), the motor assessment is symmetrical in 100% (21) of the population and all of them performed the tests for this item. In the sensory assessment, 88% (15) were present and 12% (2) absent, with 4 elderly people not having taken the assessment. When the third pair of cranial nerves was assessed, the study showed isochoric pupils in 100% (21) of the population.

The analysis of cranial nerve V (trigeminal) shows that tactile sensitivity was found in 100% (21) of the subjects, while in one subject it was not possible to carry out this analysis. Pain sensitivity was frequent in 100% of the subjects who underwent the assessment, with 4 not taking part in this item. The assessment of the mandible showed that it was present in 94% (16), while 6% (1) was absent on both sides, and this item of the research could not be carried out in 4 subjects.

As for cranial nerve pair VIII (Vestibulocochlear), hearing acuity was present in 81% (17) of the population, absent on both sides in 14% (3) and absent on one side in 5% (1). Everyone completed this item of the survey.

Still in Table 4, when we assessed the vestibular portion we found that 76% (16) had no alterations, 19% (4) had dizziness and 5% (1) reported an alteration described as the environment spinning. In the pairs of cranial nerves IX (Glossopharyngeal) and Cranial Nerves (Vagus), the voice item showed that 86% (18) had a strong, clear voice, in swallowing 95% (19) had elevation of the palate, 5% (1) had alterations and 1 subject could not be assessed.

With regard to the vomiting reflex, 88% (14) were absent and 13% (2) present, and this item could not be realised in 5 elderly people. In relation to cranial nerves XI (Accessory), muscle

muscle strength was present in 95% (19) of the population and absent on both sides in 5% (1), with one subject not having this item assessed.

As for Cranial Nerve XII (Hypoglossal), the most frequent aspect of the tongue was unchanged in 95% (20) of the population. Tongue movement was present in 100% (21) of the study subjects. Tongue strength was present in 95% (20) of the elderly studied, while speech articulation was present in 100% of the population.

Table 4 - Distribution of the results of the assessment of cranial nerve pairs of elderly residents in ILPI, Belém-Pa, 2017.

Cranial Nerve Pairs	n	%
Cranial Nerve I (Olfactory)		
Right anosmia	2	10%
Left anosmia	1	5%
Total anosmia	2	10%
Present	15	75%
Not realised	1	
Cranial Nerve II (Facial)		
Motor Assessment		
Symmetrical	21	100%
Sensory evaluation		
Absent	2	12%
Present	15	88%
Not realised	4	
Cranial Nerve III		
Isochoric	21	100%
Cranial nerve V (trigeminal)		
Tactile Sensitivity		
Present	20	100%
Not realised	1	
Pain Sensitivity		
Present	17	100%
Not realised	4	
Jaw Evaluation		
Absent (both sides)	1	6%
Present	16	94%
Not realised	4	
Cranial Nerve VIII (Vestibulocochlear)		
Hearing Acuity		
Absent	1	5%
Absent on both sides	3	14%
Present	17	81%
Vestibular Portion		
Changed: rotating environment	1	5%

No change	16	76%
Dizziness	4	19%
Cranial Nerve IX (Glossopharyngeal) Nerve and Cranial X (vagus)		
Voice		
Amended	1	5%
Changed: Weak	1	5%
Changed: low but clear	1	5%
Strong, clear sound	18	86%
Swallowing		
Changed: mushy things	1	5%
Elevation of the palate	19	95%
Not realised	1	
Vomiting reflex		
Absent	14	88%
Present	2	13%
Not realised	5	
Cranial Nerve XI (Accessory)		
Muscle strength		
Absent: two sides	1	5%
Present	19	95%
Not realised	1	
Cranial Nerve XII (Hypoglossal)		
Appearance of the tongue		
Amended	1	5%
No change	20	95%
Tongue movement		
Present	21	100%
Power of the tongue		
Absent	1	5%
Present	20	95%
Speech articulation		
Present	21	100%

Graph 1 shows the classification of blood pressure found in the study. There was a higher prevalence of normotensive patients, 38.1% (8), and 23.9% (5) of pre-hypertensive patients. 28.6% (6) had hypotension. With regard to hypertensive patients, the figure found was 4.7% (1) and only 4.7% (1) did not allow assessment.

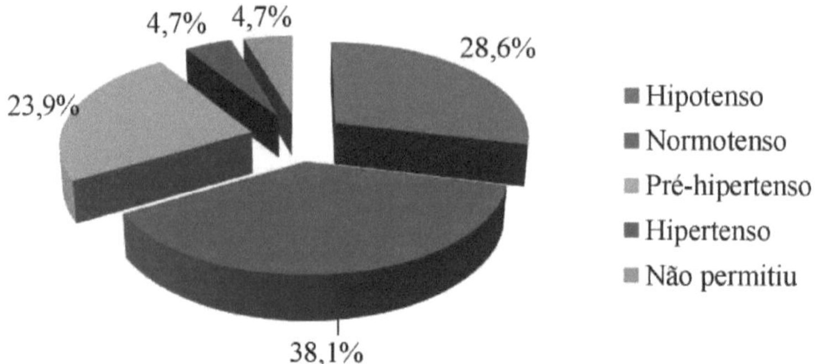

Graph 1 - Distribution of blood pressure assessment

Graph 2 shows the classification of the Body Mass Index (BMI), in which it was observed that 9.5% (2) were underweight and the same value was defended in the ideal weight 9.5% (2). With regard to the classification of overweight, 19.1% (4) were found to be obese, while grade I obesity was found in 14.3% (3), and 47.6% (10) did not undergo the assessment. This high number of elderly people who didn't undergo the assessment was due to their fear of getting on the scales.

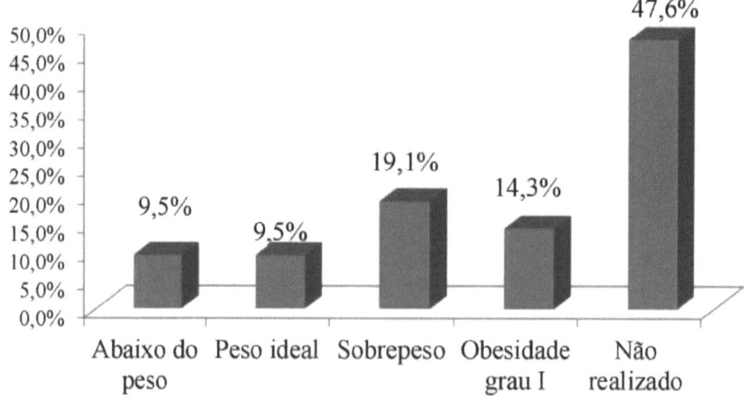

Graph 2- Distribution of the body mass index of the elderly in the study.

CHAPTER 5

DISCUSSION

In the present study, there was a higher prevalence of elderly women who were older, had no children, were retired and had lived in the ILPI for up to 10 years. This data is in line with current literature, as shown in previous studies. In the study by Silva et al. (2013), 54.8 per cent of the elderly had no children and 100 per cent received a pension. In the study by Ferreira et al. (2016), more than 50 per cent of the research subjects have been living in long-term care institutions for the elderly for more than 43 months. These data are corroborated by the study by Silva et al, (2013) which reveals a high prevalence of female elderly people with the most frequent age range between 80-89 years.

These findings reveal an increase in the life expectancy of Brazilians following the trend of demographic transition, in addition to greater investment by the public authorities in actions aimed at managing chronic conditions and consequently reducing risk factors in this population, as well as greater care and prevention of diseases (MENDES, 2011; SILVA, 2013; BRASIL, 2014).

With regard to lifestyle habits, there is a high prevalence of individuals who eat three meals, who have no dietary restrictions, who drink water frequently a day and who take part in physical activity. There is a higher frequency of chronic musculoskeletal diseases, but there is a high use of daily medication. The majority of these participants have healthy skin, use moisturisers and do not need help to carry out activities of daily living. Falls and chronic pain were frequent in this population. These findings are in line with previous studies that reveal a high rate of chronic illnesses and medication use. (2013), Guths et al., (2017), Ferreira, et al., (2016) and Oliveira, Delgado and Brascovici (2014).

With regard to chronic diseases and the use of medication, Silva, et al. (2013) showed in their study that 100% of the elderly have chronic diseases and the same number use medication. In addition, they revealed that the most prevalent diseases in their study were Diabetes Mellitus (51.6%) and Hypertension (45.2%). These results are corroborated in our research and the risk of polypharmacy in the elderly should be emphasised, as it increases the risk of side effects (SILVA, et al., 2013). In the study by Silva et al. (2017), these data are similar in parts, in which 81.3% have some type of chronic disease, but hypertension is hegemonic with 70.8%.

The results of this study, in which 81 per cent use some kind of medication, converge with those of a study by Bezerra et al. (2016) carried out with 165 elderly people in Paraíba, in which 89.3 per cent use medication (BEZERRA et al., 2016).

When it comes to the number of meals, Oliveira et al. (2014) reveal that 33.3% of the individuals in the study eat 3 meals a day and 66.6% eat 4 meals or more, which is in line with our research, which shows that 85.7% of the population eat 4 or more meals a day. A study by Benedetti et al. (2008) reported that 93.5% did not practise any type of physical activity, which is in contrast to our study, in which 66.7% practised some type of physical activity. As in the present study, Pinto et al. (2016) corroborates our findings, in which 54.6% are independent in their activities.

In the study by Guths et al. (2017), the main complaints of the participants in the research were difficulty walking and generalised pain, with 38.3% and 16.7% respectively, affirming our research regarding pain, as 66.7% had it frequently. Also in the study by Guths et al. (2017), he relates functional capacity to walking on flat terrain, and this was present in 60.1% of the population in his study, in our study we can compare it with physical activity which represents 66.7% of the population in the present study.

In the study by Ferreira, et al., (2016), which analyses the prevalence of falls in the elderly, it was shown that they occur more frequently in institutionalised elderly people than in elderly people living in the community, in addition to the majority being women living in ILPIs with less than 42 months of residence, in addition they are overweight, have a low level of physical activity and use polypharmacy. These data are in line with the present study.

When we compare the eye inspection item, our prevalence rates are 67 per cent with no alterations, which differs from studies carried out in Rio Grande do Sul, where 74.3 per cent had eye-related alterations (ROMANI, 2005).

Considering the inspection during the physical examination, we noticed that 62% of the population studied had dentures in their mouths. This fact is not in line with current literature, which shows that despite needing dentures, adherence to using them is still low. This data can be confirmed by a study carried out in João Pessoa, where only 32% of the population studied used lower dentures, while 91% of this same population needed dentures (MEDEIROS, et al., 2012).

Considering skin integrity, we realised that 67% of the individuals in the study had intact skin. This fact can be corroborated by a study carried out in Fortaleza, which suggests the main nursing diagnoses for institutionalised elderly people, among which impaired skin integrity appears in less than 18% (5) (FREITAS; PEREIRA; GUEDES, 2010).

A previous study found a high prevalence of alterations in tactile sensitivity (25%), in contrast to the present study (MALAQUIAS, et al., 2008). When analysing swallowing, only 5% were found to be altered, disagreeing with the study by Cardoso et al. (2014) in which all (100%) had altered swallowing.

An assessment of the cranial nerve pairs identified that the VIII cranial nerve pair in a study carried out in São Paulo, in three different groups of elderly people, including elderly people living in long-term care institutions, the majority had mild hearing loss (41.7%), compared to normal (25%) and moderate (33%). When we compare this with our study, in which hearing acuity was present in 81 per cent of the individuals taking part in the study, this is in disagreement with the literature (BRUNO, et al., 2016).

In relation to the 12th pair of cranial nerves (hypoglossal), a study carried out in Rio Grande do Sul showed that 60% of the population studied had normal tongue morphology, while 60% had altered tongue movement. When we relate this to our research, we can see that the morphology of the tongue can be compared to the aspect of the tongue in our study, where only 5% are altered, in disagreement with current literature. Likewise, tongue mobility can be compared with tongue movement in our study, with 100 per cent of our population having this item, which is in line with the literature presented. (OLIVEIRA, et al., 2014).

The blood pressure classification found in the study was predominantly normotensive (38.1%), which is in contrast to the study by Ferrazzo et al. (2014), where the prevalence was hypertensive with a frequency of 36%. The Body Mass Index (BMI) was more prevalent in the overweight classification, with a frequency of 19.1%. This data can be compared with a study carried out in Rio Grande do Sul which assessed the nutrition of institutionalised elderly people, revealing that 32.1% of the elderly female population was overweight **(BMI<27kg/m^2) (COLEMBERGUE**; CONDE, 2011).

CHAPTER 6

CONCLUSION

At the end of the research, we were able to observe the lifestyles, daily habits and epidemiological profile of the elderly living in a Long Stay Institution for the Elderly in Belém-Pa, as well as assessing the cranial nerve pairs, with the aim of evaluating the health conditions of this population.

In the course of the research, we were able to identify this population without children, who have lived in the ILPI studied for between 1 and 10 years, the predominant age group was between 87 and 96 years old, and all the participants in the study receive a pension.

The study also found a minority of elderly women who were sedentary, but a large part of the population had chronic diseases, particularly hypertension, diabetes and musculoskeletal disorders. During the physical examination, several alterations were identified, but most of the population had no alterations during the physical examination.

During the physical examination, the assessment of the cranial nerve pairs was highlighted by the fact that the elderly women did not agree to take part in the proposed activities; many reported fear or simply did not agree to take part in some of the cranial nerve pair assessment criteria.

The study was a great learning experience for the students and had a significant impact on the lives of the elderly participants. In order to provide better quality care, it is necessary to get to know the client in a way that takes into account various factors beyond their pathologies, and to get to know and understand the individual as a person in terms of their difficulties and daily habits.

Therefore, we can conclude that much research is still needed when it comes to the health of the elderly. The lack of acceptance of this population to take part in research is a major obstacle to overcome, but geriatric nursing has been seeking to innovate in its approach to this population, which needs special attention from health professionals, especially nurses.

CHAPTER 7

REFERENCES

ALENCAR, Mariana Asmar et al. **Profile of elderly residents in a long-stay institution.** Rev Bras Geriatr Gerontol, Rio de Janeiro, v.15, n. 4, p. 786-796. 2012.

AMANTE, Lúcia Nazareth et al. **Systematisation of nursing care in an intensive care unit based on Wanda Horta's theory.** Revista da Escola de Enfermagem da USP, São Paulo, v. 43, n. 1, p. 54-64, Oct. 2008.

BARROS; Juliana Fonseca Pontes et al. **Evaluation of the functional capacity of institutionalised elderly people in the city of Maceió - AL.** RBPS, Fortaleza, v. 23, n. 2, p. 168174, apr./jun. 2010.

BARROS, Alba Lucia Bottura Leite. **Nursing diagnosis and intervention classifications: NANDA-NIC. Acta Paulista de Enfermagem.** 22 (Especial - 70 Anos): 864-7, 2009.

BENEDETTI, Tânia Bertoldo et al. **Physical activity and mental health in the elderly.** Rev Saúde Pública. v. 42, n. 2, p. 302-7, 2008.

BEZERRA, Thaíse Alves et al. **Characterisation of medication use among elderly people treated at a basic family health unit.** Cogitare Enferm. v. 21, n. 1, p. 01-11, Jan/Mar, 2016.

BORGES, Cintia Lira et al. **Sociodemographic and clinical characteristics of institutionalised elderly: contributions to nursing care.** Rev enferm UERJ, Rio de Janeiro, v. 23, n. 3, p. 381-7, mai/jun. 2015.

BRAZIL. National Council of Health Secretaries. **Primary Care and Health Care Networks** / National Council of Health Secretaries. - Brasília: CONASS, 2015. 127 p.

BRAZIL. **Strategy for the care of people with chronic illness.** Brasilia: Ministry of Health, 2014 (Cadernos de Atenção Básica, n. 35). Available at: http://dab.saude.gov.br/portaldab/biblioteca.php?conteudo=publicacoes/cab35. Accessed on: 28 Nov. 2017.

BRUNO, Rubia Soares et al, **Auditory figure-ground ability in three different groups of elderly people.** Comin Disorders. São Paulo. v. 28. n. 1 p. 72-81. Mar, 2016

CAMARANO, Ana Amélia; KANSO, Solange. **Long-stay institutions for the elderly in Brazil.** Rev. Bras. Est. Pop, São Paulo, v. 27, n. 1, p. 233-235, jan/jun. 2010.

CARDOSO, Sabrina Vila Nova et al. **The impact of swallowing disorders on the quality of life of institutionalised elderly people.** Rev Kairós Gerontologia. v. 17, n.1, p. 232-245, March, 2014.

CARREIRA, Lígia et al. **Prevalence of depression in institutionalised elderly people.** Rev. Enferm. UERJ, Rio de Janeiro, v. 19, n. 2, p. 268- 73, Apr/Jun. 2011.

CASTRO, Vivian Carla de; CARREIRA, Lígia. **Leisure activities and attitude of institutionalised elderly people: subsidies for nursing practice.** Rev. Latino- Am. Enfermagem, Rio de Janeiro, v. 23, n. 2, p. 307-14, mar/abr. 2015.

CAUDURO, Maria Heloísa Fialho et al. **Living and health conditions of the elderly in Manaus and Porto Alegre.** Porto Alegre: EDIPUCRS, 2011. 48 p.

CAVALCANTE, Maria Ligia Silva Nunes et al. **Health indicators and the safety of institutionalised elderly people.** Rev Esc Enferm USP, São Paulo, v. 50, n. 4, p. 602-609, Jul/Aug. 2016.

CHAIMOVICZ, Flávio. **Health of the elderly.** 2. ed. Belo Horizonte: NESCON UFMG, 2013. 167 p.

CLARES, Jorge Wilker Bezerra et al. **Profile of elderly people registered at a basic family health unit in Fortaleza-ce.** Rev. Rene, Fortaleza, v. 12, n. (n. esp), p. 988-94, Apr/May 2011.

CLARES, Jorge Wilker Bezerra et al. **Systematisation of nursing care for institutionalised elderly based on Virginia Henderson.** Rev Rene, Fortaleza, v. 14, n. 3, p. *649-658,* mai/jun. 2013.

COFEN, Resolution 358/2009. **Provides for the systematisation of nursing care and the implementation of the nursing process in Brazilian health institutions,** 2009. Available at: <http://www.cofen.gov.br/resoluo-cofen- 35820094384.html> Accessed on: 14 Feb. 2016.

COMEMBERGUE, Janise Pedroso; CONDE, Simara Rufatto. **Use of the Mini Nutritional Assessment in institutionalised elderly people.** Scientia Medica. Porto Alegre. v. 21. n.2. p. 59-63. 2011.

DANTAS, Cibele Maria de Holanda Lira et al. **Functional capacity of elderly people with chronic diseases living in long-term care institutions.** Rev Bras Enferm, Brasília, v. 66, n. 6, p. 914-20, nov/dez. 2013.

DIAS, Eliane Golfieri et al. **Advanced activities of daily living as a component of the functional assessment of the elderly.** Rev Ter Ocup Univ São Paulo, São Paulo, v. 25, n. 3, p. 225-232, Sep/Dec. 2014.

DUCA, Giovâni Firpo Del et al. **Functional disability in institutionalised elderly people.** Rev Bra de Ativ Fís & Saúde, Florianópolis, v.16, n. 2, 2011.

FERRAZZO, Kívia Linhares et al. **Prehypertension, hypertension and associated factors in dental patients: a cross-sectional study in the city of Santa Maria-RS, Brazil.** Rev Odontol

UNESP. v. 43, n. 5, p. 305-313, sep/oct, 2014.

FERREIRA, Lidiane Maria de Brito Macedo et al, **Prevalence of falls and assessment of mobility in institutionalised elderly people**. Rev. Bras. Geriatr. Gerontol. Rio de Janeiro. v. 19. n.6 p. 995-1003. 2016.

FREITAS, Adriana Valéria da Silva; NORONHA, Ceci Vilar. **Elderly people in long-term care institutions: talking about care**. Interface, Botucatu, v. 1, n. 33, p. 359369, abr/jun. 2010.

FREITAS, Maria Célia de; PEREIRA, Rafaelly Fernandes; GUEDES, Maria Vilani Cavalcante. **Nursing Diagnoses in Dependent Elderly Residents of a Long-Stay Institution in Fortaleza-Ce**. Cienc. Cuid. Saude.
Fortaleza. v.8 n.3 p. 518-526. Jul/Sep 2010.

FREITAS, Mariana Gonçalves et al. **Elderly people treated in emergency services in Brazil: a study of victims of falls and road traffic accidents**. Ciên. & Saú. Colet., Rio de Janeiro, v. 20, n. 3, p.701-712, mar. 2015.

FUHRMANN, Ana Claúdia et al. **Association between the functional capacity of dependent elderly people and family carer burden**. Rev Gaúcha Enferm., Porto Alegre, v. 36, n. 1, p. 14-20, mar. 2015.

FURTADO, Luciana Gomes et al. **Nursing care for patients with sickle cell anaemia using the NHB theory and the ICNP**. Rev. RENE. Fortaleza, v.8, n.3, p 94-100, Sep/Dec.2007.

GARBACCIO, Juliana Ladeira; FERREIRA, Amanda Domingos. **Nursing diagnoses in a long-stay institution for the elderly**. R. Enferm.
Cent. O. Min, Minas Gerais, v. 2, n. 3, p. 303-313, Sep/Dec. 2012.

GOULART, Maria Stella Brandão. **The construction of change in social institutions: psychiatric reform**. Pesq. E prat. Sociais, São João del-Rei, v. 1, n. 1, jun. 2004.

GUTHS, Jucélia Fatima da Silva et al, **Sociodemographic profile, family aspects, health perceptions, functional capacity and depression in institutionalised elderly people on the North Coast of Rio Grande do Sul, Brazil**. Rev. Bras.
Geriatr. Gerontol. Rio de Janeiro, v.20. n.2 p. 175-185. 2017.

HORTA, Wanda de Aguiar. **The Nursing Process: Basis and Application**. Revista Enferm.nov. dimens, v. 1, n. 1, p. 10-6, 1975.

IBGE. 2010 Demographic Census-Distribution of **the population by sex, according to age groups**. Synopsis of the 2010 Census Results. Available at http://www.censo2010.ibge.gov.br/sinopse/webservice/. Public accessed on 30 April 2017.

LIMA, Ana et al. **Quality of life from the perspective of institutionalised elderly people.** Fortaleza CE. Rev. Bras. Promoç. Saúde, Fortaleza, v. 29, n. 1, p.14-19, jan/mar. 2016.

LIRA, Luana Nogueira et al. **Nursing diagnoses and prescriptions for elderly people in hospital.** Av. Enferm, Rio Grande do Sul, v. 33, n. 2, p. 251-260, mai/ago. 2015.

LISBOA, Cristiane Rabelo; CHIANCA, Tânia Couto Machado. **Epidemiological, clinical and functional independence profile of an institutionalised elderly population.** Rev. Bras. Enferm, Brasília, v. 65, n. 3, p. 482-7. mai/jun. 2012.

LUCCHESI, Paola Alves de Oliveira; FERRETTI-REBUSTINI, Renata Eloah de Lucena. **Nursing interventions prescribed for hospitalised elderly according to degree of dependence for Basic Activities of Daily Living.** Rev. Kair. Gerontologia, São Paulo, v. 18, n. 1, p. 199-215, jan/mar. 2015.

MACHADO, Maria de Fátima Antero Sousa et al. **Integrality, health training, health education and SUS proposals: a conceptual review.** Ciênc. saúde coletiva, Rio de Janeiro, v. 12, n. 2, mar/abr. 2007.

MALAQUIAS et al. **Risk of impaired skin integrity in hospitalised elderly people.** Cogitare Enferm. v.13, n. 3, p. 428-36, Jul/Sep, 2008.

MARCHON, Renata Marques et al. **Functional Capacity: a prospective study in elderly residents of a long-stay institution.** Rev. Bras. Geriatr. Gerontol, Rio de Janeiro, v. 13, n. 2, p. 203-214, mai/ago. 2010.

MEDEIROS, Júlia Julliêta de et al., **Edentulism, Use and Need for Prostheses and Associated Factors in a Municipality in Northeastern Brazil.** Pesq. Bras. Odontoped. Clin. Integr. João Pessoa. v. 12. n. 4. p. 573-578. oct/dec 2012.

MENDES, Eugênio Vilaça. **Health care networks.** Brasília: Pan American Health Organisation, 2011.

MENDES, Rosilda; FERNANDEZ, Juan Carlos Aneiros; SACARDO, Daniele Pompei. Health promotion and participation: approaches and questions. **Saúde debate,** Rio de Janeiro , v. 40, n. 108, p. 190-203, Mar. 2016

MIRANDA, Lívia Carvalho Viana et al. **Quality of life and associated factors in elderly people at a Reference Centre for the Elderly.** Ciên. Saúde Coletiva, v. 21, n. 11, p. 3536-3544, nov. 2016.

MORAES, Edgar Nunes de et al. **Main geriatric syndromes.** Rev Med Minas Gerais, Belo Horizonte, v. 20, n. 1, p. 54-66, 2010.

MOREIRA, Priscila de Almeida. **Quality of life of institutionalised elderly people.** 2014. 185 f. Dissertation (Master's). Federal University of Bahia, School of Nutrition,

2014.

NANDA International. NANDA Nursing Diagnoses Subtitle: Definitions and Classification 2015/2017. Artmed. 10ª edition, 2015.

OLIVEIRA, Bruna Silveira de; DELGADO, Susana Elena; BRESCOVICI, Silvana Maria. **Changes in chewing and swallowing functions in the feeding process of institutionalised elderly people.** Rev. Bras. Geriatr. Gerontol. Rio de Janeiro. v. 17. n.3 p. 575-587 2014.

OLIVEIRA, Daniel Nunes de et al. **Nursing diagnoses in elderly people in a long-stay institution.** Revista Ciência e Saúde, Porto Alegre, v. 1, n. 2, p. 57-63, jul/dez. 2008.

OLIVEIRA, Janine Melo de; ROZENDO, Célia Alves. **Long-stay institutions for the elderly: a place of care for those who have no options?** Rev. Bras. Enferm, Maceió, v. 67, n. 5, p. 773-9, Sep/Oct 2014.

OLIVEIRA, Mirna Poliana Furtado de; NOVAES, Maria Rita Carvalho Garbi. **Socioeconomic, epidemiological and pharmacotherapeutic profile of institutionalised elderly people in Brasília, Brazil.** Ciên & Saú. Coletiva, Rio de Janeiro, v. 18, n. 4, p. 1069-1078, abr. 2013.

OLIVEIRA, Roberta Rodrigues et al. **Nursing diagnoses of elderly people enrolled in family health strategies in a municipality in the interior of Goiás.** R. Enferm. Cent. O. Min, Anápolis, v. 1, n. 2, p. 248-259, Apr/Jun. 2011.

OLIVI, Maria de Lourdes; FONSECA, Rosa Maria Godoy Serpa da. **The mother under suspicion: talking about the health of school-age children.** Revista da Escola de Enfermagem USP, São Paulo, v. 41, n. 2, p. 213-21, 2007.

PEREIRA, Lilian et al. **Pain intensity in institutionalised elderly: comparison between numerical scales and verbal descriptors.** Rev Esc Enferm USP, Goiânia, v. 49, n. 5, p.804-810, 2015.

PINHEIRO, Natália Cristina Garcia et al. **Inequality in the profile of institutionalised elderly people in the city of Natal, Brazil.** Ciênc. Saúde Coletiva, Rio de Janeiro, v. 21, n. 11, p. 3399- 3405, nov. 2016.

PINTO, Andressa Hoffmann et al. **Functional capacity for activities of daily living of elderly people from the Family Health Strategy in rural areas.** Ciência & Saúde Coletiva. V. 21, p. 11, p. 3545-3555, 2016

PIRES, Laurena Moreira et al. **Nursing in the context of schoolchildren's health: Integrative literature review.** Revista de Enfermagem UERJ, Rio de Janeiro, v. 20, n. 5, p. 668-675, dec. 2013.

POLARO, Sandra Helen Isse et al. **Elderly residents in long-stay institutions for the elderly in the metropolitan region of Belém-PA.** Rev. Bras. Geriatr. Gerontol, Rio de

Janeiro, v. 15, n.4, p. 777-784, Oct/Dec. 2012.

ROMANI, Flávio Antonio. **Prevalence of ocular disorders in the elderly population living in the city of Veranópolis**, RS, Brazil. Arq Bras Oftalmol. v. 68, n. 5, p. 649-55, 2005.

ROSA, Tábada Samantha Marques et al. **The institutionalised elderly: sociodemographic and clinical-functional profiles related to dizziness.** Braz J Otorhinolaryngol, São Paulo, v. 82, n. 2, p. 159-169, mar/abr. 2016.

SANTOS, Jênifa Cavalcante dos et al. **Elderly adherence to treatment for arterial hypertension and nursing interventions.** Rev. Rene, Fortaleza, v. 13, n. 2, p. 343-53, 2012.

SILVA, Amanda Ramalho et al. **Chronic non-communicable diseases and sociodemographic factors associated with symptoms of depression in the elderly.** J Bras Psiquiatr. v. 66, n. 1, p. 45-51, 2017.

SILVA, Bárbara; SANTOS, Silvana. **Care for the institutionalised elderly - opinions of the nurse collective subject for 2016.** Acta Paul Enferm, Rio Grande, v. 23, n. 6, p. 775-781, 2010.

SILVA, Luiz Anildo Anacleto da et al. **Permanent education in health and nursing work: the perspective of a transforming praxis.** Rev. Gaúcha de Enferm, Porto Alegre, v. 31, n. 3, p. 557-61, Sep. 2010.

SILVA, Malu Emanuelle et al, **Epidemiological, sociodemographic and clinical profile of institutionalised elderly people.** R. Enferm. Cent. O. Minas Gerais. v. 3 n.1 p. 569-576. 2013.

SILVA, Norhan Sumar et al. **Sistematização da assistência de enfermagem em saúde da família sob a óptica de enfermeiros de Petrópolis - RJ.** Rev. Pesq : cuid. fundam., Rio de Janeiros, 2(Ed. Supl.), p. 657-660, Oct/Dec. 2010.

SMANIOTO, Franciele Nogueira; HADDAD, Maria do Carmo Fernandez Lourenço. **Katz index applied to institutionalised elderly.** Rev Rene, Fortaleza, v. 12, n. 1, p. 18-23, jan/mar. 2011.

SOARES, Cristiane Bárbara et al. **Emancipatory action research: an essential methodological proposal for nursing.** In: National Seminar on Nursing Research, 17, 2013 Jun3-5. Proceedings. Natal: Brazilian Nursing Association - Rio Grande do Norte Section, 2013.

SUDRÉ, Mayara Rocha Siqueira et al. **Socioeconomic and health characteristics of elderly people assisted by family health teams.** Cienc Cuid Saude, Cuiabá, v. 14, n. 1, p. 933-940, jan/mar. 2014.

TEIXEIRA, Mima Barros et al. **Evaluation of health promotion practices: a look at the** teams participating in the National Programme for Improving Primary Care Access and Quality. Saúde debate, Rio de Janeiro, v. 38. n. especial, p. 5268, oct. 2014.

TOLEDO, Renata Ferraz de et al. **Action research in interdisciplinary studies: analysing criteria that only practice can reveal.** Interface, Botucatu, v. 18, n. 51, p. 633-646, sep. 2014.

VARELA, Gisele de Castro et al. **Systematisation of Nursing Care in the Family Health Strategy: Limits and Possibilities.** Revista Rene, v. 13, n. 4, p. 816-24, Sep/Dec. 2012.

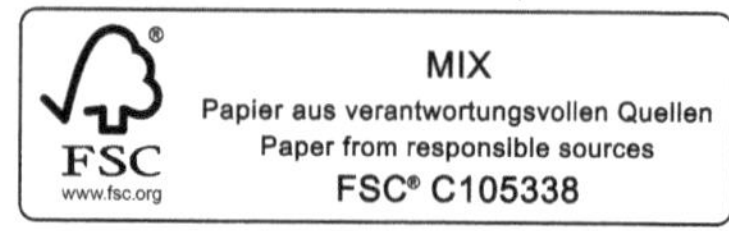

Printed by Books on Demand GmbH, Norderstedt / Germany